Nutrition and Cancer Prevention: A Comprehensive Guide to a Cancer-Free Diet

Bob Philz.

Table Of Contents

Introduction: The Power of Nutrition in Cancer Prevention

Cancer is one of the leading causes of death worldwide, but a significant portion of cancer cases can be prevented through lifestyle and dietary choices. In "Nutrition and Cancer Prevention: A Comprehensive Guide to a Cancer-Free Diet," we will explore the profound impact that nutrition has on cancer risk and how you can harness the power of food to protect yourself and your loved ones. This book is designed to be a practical, evidence-based resource, providing you with the knowledge and tools to make informed dietary choices that can lower your risk of cancer.

By understanding the science behind cancer and nutrition, incorporating anti-cancer foods into your diet, and adopting healthy eating habits, you can take proactive steps toward a healthier, cancer-free life. Let's embark on this journey together and discover how the right nutrition can be your strongest ally in the fight against cancer.

Understanding Cancer: An Overview

Cancer is a complex group of diseases characterized by the uncontrolled growth and spread of abnormal cells. If the spread is not controlled, it can result in death. Cancer can affect almost any part of the body, and the causes are multifactorial, including genetic predispositions, environmental exposures, and lifestyle choices.

There are more than 100 types of cancer, each classified by the type of cell that is initially affected. For example, carcinoma originates in the skin or tissues that line or cover internal organs, while sarcoma begins in bone, cartilage, fat, muscle, blood vessels, or other connective or supportive tissue. Leukemia starts in blood-forming tissue such as the bone marrow and results in large numbers of abnormal blood cells being produced and entering the blood. Lymphoma and myeloma are cancers that begin in the cells of the immune system.

The process of carcinogenesis, or the development of cancer, involves multiple stages: initiation, promotion, and progression. During initiation, genetic damage or mutations occur. Promotion involves the proliferation of these damaged cells, and progression leads to the formation of tumors and the potential spread of cancer to other parts of the body (metastasis).

The Role of Diet in Health and Disease

Diet is a cornerstone of health, influencing a myriad of bodily functions and playing a crucial role in the prevention and management of many diseases, including cancer. The foods we consume provide essential nutrients that are necessary for the body's maintenance, growth, and repair. A healthy diet supports the immune system, helps maintain a healthy weight, and reduces the risk of chronic diseases.

Conversely, poor dietary choices can lead to nutrient deficiencies, obesity, and increased susceptibility to various diseases. Obesity, in particular, is a significant risk factor for several types of cancer, including breast, colorectal, endometrial, and esophageal cancers. Diets high in processed foods, red and processed meats, and sugary beverages contribute to inflammation, insulin resistance, and hormonal imbalances, which can promote the development of cancer.

The Link Between Nutrition and Cancer

The relationship between nutrition and cancer is complex and multifaceted. Nutrients and bioactive compounds in foods can influence carcinogenesis through various mechanisms, including antioxidant activity, modulation of detoxification enzymes, immune function enhancement, and anti-inflammatory effects.

- **Antioxidants:** Antioxidants such as vitamins C and E, selenium, and beta-carotene help neutralize free radicals—unstable molecules that can damage cells and contribute to cancer development. By preventing oxidative stress, antioxidants protect cellular integrity and function.

- **Phytochemicals:** These are naturally occurring compounds found in plants that have protective effects against cancer. Examples include flavonoids, carotenoids, and polyphenols. Phytochemicals can inhibit cancer cell proliferation, induce apoptosis (programmed cell death), and prevent angiogenesis (the formation of new blood vessels that feed tumors).

- **Fiber:** Dietary fiber, found in whole grains, fruits, vegetables, and legumes, plays a critical role in maintaining a healthy digestive system. Fiber aids in the removal of carcinogens from the gastrointestinal tract and promotes regular bowel movements, reducing the risk of colorectal cancer.

Numerous studies have demonstrated the protective effects of a diet rich in fruits, vegetables, whole grains, and lean proteins. For instance, the EPIC (European Prospective Investigation into Cancer and Nutrition) study highlighted that high intakes of fruits, vegetables, and fiber are associated with a reduced risk of colorectal cancer. Similarly, the Nurses' Health Study and Health

Professionals Follow-Up Study found that high consumption of red and processed meats is linked to an increased risk of colorectal cancer, while diets rich in fruits and vegetables are associated with a lower risk of breast and other cancers.

The impact of specific foods and nutrients on cancer prevention has been extensively studied:

- **Fruits and Vegetables:** These are rich in vitamins, minerals, fiber, and phytochemicals. Consuming a variety of colorful fruits and vegetables ensures a wide range of beneficial nutrients that can protect against different types of cancer.

- **Whole Grains:** Whole grains such as brown rice, quinoa, oats, and whole wheat provide dietary fiber, vitamins, and minerals. Fiber, in particular, promotes digestive health and may reduce the risk of colorectal cancer.

- **Nuts and Seeds:** Nuts and seeds are packed with healthy fats, protein, and essential nutrients. They contain phytochemicals and antioxidants that protect against cellular damage.

- **Healthy Fats:** Omega-3 fatty acids, found in fatty fish, flaxseeds, chia seeds, and walnuts, have anti-inflammatory and cancer-preventive properties. Maintaining a balance between omega-3 and omega-6 fatty acids is crucial for reducing cancer risk.

Understanding the power of nutrition in cancer prevention allows individuals to make informed dietary choices that can significantly reduce their risk of developing cancer. By adopting a diet rich in whole, plant-based foods and minimizing the intake of processed and high-sugar foods, we can harness the protective benefits of nutrition to promote long-term health and well-being.

In this book, we will delve deeper into the specific foods and nutrients that have been shown to prevent cancer, explore practical tips for incorporating them into your daily diet, and provide you with the knowledge and tools to create a cancer-preventive dietary plan. Let's embark on this journey towards a healthier, cancer-free life by harnessing the power of nutrition.

Chapter 1: The Science Behind Cancer and Nutrition

How Cancer Develops: An Insight into Carcinogenesis

Cancer development, known as carcinogenesis, is a multi-step process involving genetic mutations and cellular transformations. The stages of carcinogenesis include initiation, promotion, and progression.

Cancer begins when cells in the body start to grow uncontrollably. Normally, human cells grow and divide to form new cells as the body needs them. When cells grow old or become damaged, they die, and new cells take their place. However, when cancer develops, this orderly process breaks down. Cells become increasingly abnormal, old or damaged cells survive when they should die, and new cells form when they are not needed. These extra cells can divide without stopping and may form growths called tumors.

Carcinogenesis, the process of developing cancer, is influenced by genetic mutations and environmental factors. These mutations can be inherited, induced by exposure to carcinogens, or occur randomly. A combination of multiple mutations can lead to uncontrolled cell growth, resulting in cancer.

The stages of cancer development can be clsassified as follows:

- **Initiation:** This stage involves genetic mutations that occur due to exposure to carcinogens (e.g., tobacco smoke, radiation, certain chemicals) or inherited genetic factors. These mutations alter the normal functioning of genes responsible for cell growth and division.
- **Promotion:** During this phase, the initiated cells begin to proliferate abnormally. Promoting agents, which may include certain hormones or dietary components, encourage the growth of these mutated cells. Unlike the initiation phase, the promotion phase is potentially reversible if

the promoting agents are removed or countered by protective factors.

- **Progression:** This final stage involves the further growth and spread of the abnormal cells, leading to the formation of malignant tumors. These tumors can invade surrounding tissues and metastasize to other parts of the body through the bloodstream or lymphatic system.

The process of carcinogenesis is influenced by a variety of factors, including genetic predisposition, environmental exposures, and lifestyle choices. Understanding these factors and their interactions is crucial for developing effective cancer prevention strategies.

Nutritional Science: How Diet Influences Cancer Risk

Nutrition plays a pivotal role in modifying the risk of cancer. Certain dietary patterns and nutrients can either promote or inhibit carcinogenesis. For instance, diets high in fruits, vegetables, and whole grains are associated with a lower risk of several types of cancer, while diets high in red and processed meats, sugary beverages, and refined grains are linked to an increased risk.

Diet plays a pivotal role in either promoting or protecting against cancer. The foods we consume contain a variety of compounds that can influence cellular processes, including those involved in carcinogenesis. Nutrients and bioactive compounds in foods can influence carcinogenesis through various mechanisms:

Protective Nutrients and Compounds:

Antioxidants: Compounds such as vitamins C and E, selenium, and carotenoids can neutralize free radicals, preventing cellular damage. Free radicals are unstable molecules that can damage DNA, proteins, and cell membranes, leading to cancer development.

Phytochemicals: Found in plants, these compounds can inhibit cancer cell proliferation, induce apoptosis (programmed cell death), and hinder angiogenesis (formation of new blood vessels that feed tumors).

These plant-based compounds, including flavonoids, carotenoids, and polyphenols, have anti-carcinogenic properties. They can inhibit cancer cell proliferation, induce apoptosis (programmed cell death), and block angiogenesis (the formation of new blood vessels that supply tumors).

Fiber: Dietary fiber promotes a healthy digestive system and may reduce the risk of colorectal cancer.

Dietary fiber, found in whole grains, fruits, vegetables, and legumes, helps maintain a healthy digestive system. It promotes regular bowel movements and may bind to carcinogens, facilitating their removal from the body.

Risk-Promoting Nutrients and Compounds:

Processed Meats: Consumption of processed meats, such as sausages and bacon, has been linked to an increased risk of colorectal cancer. These meats often contain nitrates and nitrites, which can form carcinogenic compounds during digestion.

Red Meat: High intake of red meat, particularly when cooked at high temperatures (e.g., grilling or frying), can lead to the formation of carcinogenic compounds like heterocyclic amines and polycyclic aromatic hydrocarbons.

Sugary Foods and Beverages: Diets high in sugar can lead to obesity and insulin resistance, both of which are risk factors for several types of cancer, including breast, colorectal, and endometrial cancers.

Key Studies and Breakthroughs in Cancer Nutrition Research

Over the years, numerous studies have provided evidence linking diet to cancer risk. Research has continually highlighted the impact of diet on cancer prevention. Some landmark studies include:

The EPIC Study (European Prospective Investigation into Cancer and Nutrition):

This large-scale study has followed over half a million participants across 10 European countries. It has provided extensive data on the relationship between diet and cancer. Findings indicate that high intakes of fruits, vegetables, and fiber are associated with a reduced risk of colorectal cancer. Additionally, the study has highlighted the risks associated with high consumption of red and processed meats.

This study has provided extensive data showing that a diet rich in fruits, vegetables, and fiber is associated with a reduced risk of colorectal and other cancers.

The Nurses' Health Study and Health Professionals Follow-Up Study:

These long-term studies have followed large cohorts of nurses and health professionals in the United States. Research from these studies has shown that diets high in red and processed meats are linked to an increased risk of colorectal cancer, while high intakes of fruits and vegetables are associated with a lower risk of breast and other cancers. The studies have also provided insights into the role of dietary fats, showing that a high intake of trans fats is associated with an increased risk of breast cancer.

The Adventist Health Studies:

Conducted among Seventh-day Adventists, these studies have highlighted the benefits of a plant-based diet. Findings suggest that vegetarians and vegans have a lower risk of several types of cancer compared to non-vegetarians. Studies have also shown that high consumption of nuts and soy products is associated with a reduced risk of certain cancers.

The China-Cornell-Oxford Project (China Study):

This comprehensive study examined the dietary habits of different populations in China and their association with disease prevalence. The research found that diets high in animal products and low in plant-based foods are linked to increased cancer rates, while diets rich in fruits, vegetables, and whole grains are protective.

These key studies and many others have provided robust evidence supporting the role of diet in cancer prevention. They highlight the importance of a balanced diet rich in fruits, vegetables, whole grains, and lean proteins, while minimizing the intake of processed foods, red and processed meats, and sugary beverages.

The body of research underscores the significance of dietary choices in modulating cancer risk. By understanding and applying these findings, individuals can take proactive steps to reduce their cancer risk through informed nutritional practices.

Chapter 2: Anti-Cancer Foods: What to Eat and Why

Fruits and Vegetables: Nature's Protective Shield

Fruits and vegetables are essential components of a cancer-preventive diet due to their high content of vitamins, minerals, fiber, and a diverse array of phytochemicals. These foods provide the body with the necessary nutrients to maintain cellular health, boost the immune system, and protect against oxidative stress and inflammation, which are key factors in cancer development.

Fruits and vegetables are particularly rich in antioxidants, which neutralize free radicals, preventing them from causing cellular damage that can lead to cancer. Additionally, the fiber in fruits and vegetables aids in digestion, helps regulate blood sugar levels, and supports a healthy gut microbiome, all of which contribute to reduced cancer risk.

Cruciferous Vegetables: Broccoli, Cauliflower, and Brussels Sprouts

Cruciferous vegetables, such as broccoli, cauliflower, and Brussels sprouts, are known for their potent anti-cancer properties. These vegetables contain glucosinolates, sulfur-containing compounds that, when broken down, form biologically active compounds like indoles, nitriles, thiocyanates, and isothiocyanates. These compounds have been shown to inhibit the development of cancer in several organs in rats and mice, including the bladder, breast, colon, liver, lung, and stomach.

Broccoli: This vegetable is rich in sulforaphane, an isothiocyanate that has been extensively studied for its cancer-fighting properties. Sulforaphane can inhibit the growth of cancer cells, promote their death, and enhance the detoxification of carcinogens.

Cauliflower: Like broccoli, cauliflower contains glucosinolates and isothiocyanates that help protect against cancer by reducing inflammation, neutralizing toxins, and preventing the spread of cancer cells.

Brussels Sprouts: These are packed with fiber, vitamins C and K, and folate, along with glucosinolates that convert to cancer-protective compounds.

Berries: Blueberries, Strawberries, and Raspberries

Berries are among the most nutrient-dense fruits and are particularly rich in antioxidants, vitamins, and fiber. They contain high levels of anthocyanins, ellagic acid, and other phytochemicals that have been shown to have anti-cancer properties.

Blueberries: These are rich in anthocyanins and resveratrol, which have strong antioxidant and anti-inflammatory effects. Studies have shown that blueberry extracts can inhibit the growth of cancer cells and reduce the risk of several types of cancer, including breast, colon, and prostate cancer.

Strawberries: Strawberries are high in vitamin C, manganese, and fiber, and contain ellagic acid, which has been shown to prevent skin, bladder, lung, esophagus, and breast cancers.

Raspberries: These are packed with vitamins, minerals, and ellagic acid. They have been found to inhibit cancer cell growth and prevent the formation of blood vessels that supply tumors.

Whole Grains: The Importance of Fiber

Whole grains, such as brown rice, quinoa, oats, and whole wheat, are important sources of dietary fiber, vitamins, minerals, and phytonutrients. The consumption of whole grains has been linked to a reduced risk of several types of cancer, particularly colorectal cancer.

Fiber: Dietary fiber helps maintain a healthy digestive system by promoting regular bowel movements and preventing constipation. It also helps in the removal of carcinogens from the gastrointestinal tract. Additionally, fiber can regulate blood sugar levels and support a healthy weight, both of which are important for cancer prevention.

Phytochemicals: Whole grains contain lignans, phenolic acids, and other phytonutrients that have antioxidant and anti-inflammatory properties. These compounds can protect cells from damage, reduce inflammation, and inhibit the growth of cancer cells.

Nuts and Seeds: Small but Mighty

Nuts and seeds are nutrient-dense foods that provide healthy fats, protein, fiber, vitamins, minerals, and a variety of phytochemicals. They have been associated with a reduced risk of several types of cancer, including colorectal, endometrial, and pancreatic cancers.

Almonds: Rich in vitamin E, magnesium, and healthy fats, almonds can protect against oxidative stress and inflammation, reducing cancer risk.

Walnuts: These contain high levels of omega-3 fatty acids, polyphenols, and phytosterols, all of which have anti-cancer properties. Walnuts have been shown to slow the growth of breast and prostate cancer cells.

Flaxseeds and Chia Seeds: These are excellent sources of omega-3 fatty acids, lignans, and fiber. Omega-3s have anti-inflammatory effects, while lignans can inhibit the growth of hormone-related cancers, such as breast and prostate cancer.

Legumes: Beans, Lentils, and Peas

Legumes, including beans, lentils, and peas, are rich in protein, fiber, vitamins, and minerals. They also contain a variety of bioactive compounds, such as saponins, protease inhibitors, and phytic acid, which have been shown to have anti-cancer properties.

Beans: Black beans, kidney beans, and navy beans are high in fiber, protein, and antioxidants. They can help regulate blood sugar levels, support a healthy gut microbiome, and reduce the risk of colorectal cancer.

Lentils: These are a great source of folate, iron, and polyphenols. Lentils have been shown to inhibit the growth of cancer cells and reduce the risk of several types of cancer.

Peas: Green peas and split peas are rich in fiber, protein, and vitamins. They contain compounds that can inhibit cancer cell proliferation and support overall health.

By incorporating a variety of these anti-cancer foods into your diet, you can harness their protective benefits to reduce your risk of cancer and promote overall health. Aim to fill your plate with a rainbow of fruits and vegetables, choose whole grains over refined grains, enjoy nuts and seeds as snacks or additions to meals, and include legumes as a regular part of your diet. These foods, with their diverse and powerful nutrients, provide a strong defense against cancer and support a healthy, vibrant lifestyle.

Chapter 3: Powerful Phytochemicals and Antioxidants

Understanding Phytochemicals: Nature's Defense Compounds

Phytochemicals, also known as phytonutrients, are naturally occurring compounds found in plants that provide a variety of health benefits. These bioactive compounds are responsible for the color, flavor, and aroma of fruits and vegetables. They have been extensively studied for their role in disease prevention, particularly in cancer prevention.

Phytochemicals can influence various biological processes in the body, helping to protect against cellular damage, inflammation, and the development of chronic diseases. They work through several mechanisms, including antioxidant activity, modulation of detoxification enzymes, stimulation of the immune system, and alteration of hormone metabolism.

There are thousands of phytochemicals, but some of the most well-known and studied include flavonoids, carotenoids, glucosinolates, and polyphenols. Each type of phytochemical has unique properties and contributes to health in different ways.

Key Antioxidants and Their Role in Cancer Prevention

Antioxidants are compounds that protect cells from damage caused by free radicals—unstable molecules that can harm cellular structures. Free radicals are generated naturally in the body during metabolic processes and can also be introduced through external sources like pollution, radiation, and tobacco smoke. When free radicals accumulate, they can cause oxidative stress, leading to cellular damage and increasing the risk of chronic diseases, including cancer.

Several antioxidants play a crucial role in neutralizing free radicals and protecting cells:

Vitamins C and E: These vitamins are powerful antioxidants that help protect cells from oxidative damage. Vitamin C is water-soluble and can regenerate other antioxidants, while vitamin E is fat-soluble and protects cell membranes from lipid peroxidation.

Selenium: This trace mineral is an essential component of antioxidant enzymes, such as glutathione peroxidase, which helps neutralize harmful peroxides in the body. Selenium also supports the immune system and has been shown to reduce the risk of certain cancers.

Beta-carotene: This carotenoid is a precursor to vitamin A and is found in colorful fruits and vegetables. It has antioxidant properties and can enhance immune function and protect against cellular damage.

Vitamins C and E, Selenium, and Beta-Carotene

Vitamin C: Also known as ascorbic acid, vitamin C is found in high concentrations in fruits and vegetables, particularly citrus fruits, strawberries, bell peppers, and broccoli. It plays a vital role in collagen synthesis, wound healing, and the maintenance of healthy skin, blood vessels, and bones. Vitamin C also enhances the absorption of iron from plant-based foods and supports the immune system.

Vitamin E: This fat-soluble vitamin exists in eight different forms, with alpha-tocopherol being the most biologically active in humans. Vitamin E is abundant in nuts, seeds, and vegetable oils, as well as in green leafy vegetables. It acts as a potent antioxidant, protecting cell membranes from oxidative damage. Vitamin E also plays a role in immune function and skin health.

Selenium: Selenium is a trace mineral found in soil, and its content in foods can vary depending on the soil where they were grown. Rich dietary sources of selenium include Brazil nuts, seafood, and organ meats. Selenium is crucial for the proper functioning of antioxidant enzymes and supports thyroid health and immune function.

Beta-Carotene: This carotenoid is converted into vitamin A in the body and is found in orange and yellow fruits and vegetables, such as carrots, sweet potatoes, and mangoes, as well as in leafy greens like spinach and kale. Beta-carotene has antioxidant properties and supports vision, immune function, and skin health.

Top Sources of Phytochemicals and How to Incorporate Them into Your Diet

Incorporating a wide variety of phytochemical-rich foods into your diet can help reduce cancer risk and promote overall health. Here are some top sources of key phytochemicals and practical tips on how to include them in your meals:

Flavonoids:

Sources: Apples, onions, dark chocolate, tea (especially green tea), berries, and citrus fruits.

Incorporation: Enjoy a cup of green tea with breakfast, snack on apples or berries, and add onions to salads, soups, and stir-fries.

Carotenoids:

Sources: Carrots, sweet potatoes, tomatoes, spinach, kale, and bell peppers.

Incorporation: Make a colorful vegetable stir-fry, blend a smoothie with spinach and mango, or add roasted carrots and sweet potatoes as a side dish.

Glucosinolates:

Sources: Broccoli, Brussels sprouts, cauliflower, cabbage, and kale.

Incorporation: Steam or roast cruciferous vegetables as a side dish, add raw kale to salads or blend cauliflower into soups and smoothies for added creaminess.

Polyphenols:

Sources: Berries, cherries, grapes, nuts, seeds, and dark chocolate.

Incorporation: Top yogurt or oatmeal with a mix of berries, snack on a handful of nuts and seeds, and enjoy a small piece of dark chocolate as a treat.

Lignans:

Sources: Flaxseeds, sesame seeds, whole grains, and vegetables.

Incorporation: Add ground flaxseeds to smoothies, yogurt, or oatmeal, sprinkle sesame seeds on salads, and choose whole-grain bread and cereals.

Saponins:

Sources: Legumes, such as beans, lentils, and chickpeas.

Incorporation: Include legumes in soups, stews, salads, and dips like hummus.

To maximize the benefits of phytochemicals and antioxidants, aim to consume a diverse range of plant-based foods daily. Experiment with new recipes and cooking methods to keep your meals interesting and flavorful. By making these nutrient-rich foods a regular part of your diet, you can harness their protective effects to reduce your risk of cancer and enhance your overall health and well-being.

Understanding the science behind phytochemicals and antioxidants, recognizing their sources, and incorporating them into your diet can significantly contribute to cancer prevention and a healthier life.

Chapter 4: The Role of Healthy Fats in Cancer Prevention

Omega-3 Fatty Acids: Benefits and Sources

Omega-3 fatty acids are essential polyunsaturated fats that play a crucial role in maintaining overall health and preventing chronic diseases, including cancer. These fats are termed "essential" because the body cannot produce them on its own; therefore, they must be obtained through diet. Omega-3 fatty acids are known for their anti-inflammatory properties, which are significant in cancer prevention since chronic inflammation is a well-established risk factor for cancer development.

Benefits of Omega-3 Fatty Acids:

Anti-Inflammatory Properties: Omega-3 fatty acids help reduce inflammation by modulating inflammatory pathways. This is particularly important because chronic inflammation can lead to DNA damage, promote tumor growth, and support the spread of cancer cells.

Cell Membrane Health: These fatty acids are integral components of cell membranes, enhancing cell fluidity and communication, which are vital for maintaining cellular function and preventing mutations.

Immune System Support: Omega-3s help regulate immune responses, ensuring that the body can effectively target and destroy abnormal cells before they become cancerous.

Inhibition of Tumor Growth: Research suggests that omega-3 fatty acids can inhibit the growth of various cancer cells, including breast, prostate, and colorectal cancers, by inducing apoptosis (programmed cell death) and reducing angiogenesis (the formation of new blood vessels that supply tumors).

Sources of Omega-3 Fatty Acids:

Fatty Fish: Salmon, mackerel, sardines, and trout are excellent sources of eicosapentaenoic acid (EPA) and docosahexaenoic acid (DHA), two long-chain omega-3 fatty acids.

Flaxseeds: These are rich in alpha-linolenic acid (ALA), a plant-based omega-3 fatty acid. Ground flaxseeds can be added to smoothies, oatmeal, or baked goods.

Chia Seeds: Another great source of ALA, chia seeds can be sprinkled on yogurt, salads, or incorporated into puddings.

Walnuts: These nuts provide a good amount of ALA and make for a convenient snack or addition to various dishes.

Algal Oil: This plant-based supplement is derived from algae and provides DHA, making it a suitable option for vegetarians and vegans.

The Balance Between Omega-6 and Omega-3 Fatty Acids

Maintaining a proper balance between omega-6 and omega-3 fatty acids is crucial for optimal health and cancer prevention. Both types of fatty acids are essential, but the typical Western diet tends to be disproportionately high in omega-6s and low in omega-3s. This imbalance can promote inflammation and increase cancer risk.

Understanding Omega-6 Fatty Acids:

Omega-6 fatty acids, found in vegetable oils like corn, soybean, and sunflower oils, as well as in processed foods, play a role in inflammatory responses, blood clotting, and cell proliferation.

While *omega-6s* are necessary for health, excessive intake without adequate omega-3s can lead to an pro-inflammatory state.

Ideal Omega-6 to Omega-3 Ratio:

- Historically, humans consumed omega-6 and omega-3 fatty acids in a ratio of approximately 1:1 to 4:1. However, the modern diet often features ratios as high as 20:1 or more.
- Striving for a balanced ratio (closer to 4:1) can help reduce inflammation and lower the risk of chronic diseases, including cancer.

Tips for Achieving Balance:

Increase Omega-3 Intake: Incorporate more omega-3-rich foods into your diet, such as fatty fish, flaxseeds, chia seeds, and walnuts.

Reduce Omega-6 Intake: Limit consumption of processed foods and oils high in omega-6 fatty acids. Opt for healthier cooking oils, such as olive oil or avocado oil, which have a more favorable fatty acid profile.

Choose Whole Foods: Emphasize whole, unprocessed foods in your diet to naturally balance your intake of essential fatty acids.

Healthy Fat Sources: Fish, Flaxseeds, Chia Seeds, and Nuts

Incorporating a variety of healthy fat sources into your diet can provide the necessary nutrients for cancer prevention and overall health. Here's how you can effectively include these foods:

Fatty Fish:

- **Salmon:** Rich in EPA and DHA, salmon can be baked, grilled, or added to salads for a nutritious meal.
- **Mackerel and Sardines:** These fish are also high in omega-3s and can be enjoyed fresh, canned, or smoked. They are convenient options for quick meals or snacks.

Flaxseeds:

- **Ground Flaxseeds:** Whole flaxseeds can pass through the digestive system undigested, so it's best to consume them ground to absorb their nutrients. Add ground flaxseeds to smoothies, oatmeal, or yogurt.
- **Flaxseed Oil:** This oil can be used in salad dressings or drizzled over vegetables. However, it should not be heated, as high temperatures can destroy its beneficial properties.

Chia Seeds:

- **Chia Pudding:** Mix chia seeds with your choice of milk (dairy or plant-based) and let them sit overnight to create a nutritious pudding.
- **Smoothie Add-In:** Blend chia seeds into your smoothies for an extra boost of omega-3s and fiber.

Nuts:

- **Walnuts:** Enjoy walnuts as a snack, add them to salads, or incorporate them into baked goods for a crunchy texture and nutritional benefits.
- **Almonds and Pistachios:** While not as high in omega-3s, these nuts are still excellent sources of healthy fats, protein, and fiber. They can be included in a variety of dishes or enjoyed on their own.

Algal Oil:

- **Supplements**: Algal oil supplements are available for those who may not consume enough omega-3s from dietary sources, particularly for vegetarians and vegans. These supplements provide a direct source of DHA.

Healthy fats, particularly omega-3 fatty acids, play a significant role in cancer prevention. By understanding their benefits, maintaining a balanced intake of omega-6 and omega-3 fatty acids, and incorporating a variety of nutrient-rich fat sources into your diet, you can support overall health and reduce your risk of cancer. Making these dietary adjustments can have a profound impact on your well-being and longevity.

Chapter 5: The Impact of Sugar and Processed Foods

How Sugar Feeds Cancer Cells

The relationship between sugar and cancer has been a topic of considerable research and debate. While sugar itself does not directly cause cancer, its consumption can contribute to an environment in the body that supports cancer growth and development. Here's how:

Insulin Resistance and Hyperinsulinemia:

Insulin Resistance: High sugar intake can lead to insulin resistance, where the body's cells become less responsive to insulin. This condition forces the pancreas to produce more insulin to maintain normal blood glucose levels.

Hyperinsulinemia: Chronically elevated insulin levels (hyperinsulinemia) are associated with an increased risk of certain cancers. Insulin is a growth-promoting hormone, and high levels can stimulate the proliferation of cancer cells and inhibit apoptosis (programmed cell death).

Inflammation:

Excessive sugar consumption can lead to chronic inflammation, a known risk factor for cancer. High blood glucose levels can cause oxidative stress, leading to the production of inflammatory cytokines and creating a pro-inflammatory state conducive to cancer development.

Obesity:

Diets high in sugar and refined carbohydrates contribute to weight gain and obesity, which are major risk factors for various cancers. Adipose tissue (body fat) produces hormones and inflammatory molecules that can promote cancer cell growth and progression.

Cancer Metabolism:

Cancer cells have a high demand for glucose to fuel their rapid growth and division. This phenomenon, known as the "Warburg effect," describes how cancer cells preferentially use glycolysis (a less efficient form of energy production) even in the presence of oxygen. High blood sugar levels can provide the necessary fuel for these rapidly proliferating cells.

The Risks of Processed and Ultra-Processed Foods

Processed and *ultra-processed* foods are increasingly prevalent in modern diets, but their consumption is linked to numerous health risks, including cancer. These foods are typically high in unhealthy fats, sugars, and additives, and low in essential nutrients.

Processed Foods:

Definition: Foods that have been altered from their natural state for preservation or convenience, including canned vegetables, cheeses, and packaged meats.

Risks: Processed foods often contain added sugars, unhealthy fats, and sodium, which can contribute to inflammation, insulin resistance, and obesity—all risk factors for cancer.

Ultra-Processed Foods:

Definition: Industrial formulations made mostly from substances extracted from foods (e.g., oils, fats, sugar, starch, and proteins) and additives, including sweeteners, flavor enhancers, colorants, emulsifiers, and preservatives. Examples include sugary beverages, packaged snacks, instant noodles, and ready-to-eat meals.

Risks: Ultra-processed foods are typically energy-dense and nutrient-poor, leading to overconsumption of calories and insufficient intake of essential nutrients. They often contain artificial ingredients that may have carcinogenic properties. Regular consumption of these foods is linked to increased risks of obesity, diabetes, and cancers such as colorectal, breast, and prostate cancer.

Strategies to Reduce Sugar and Processed Food Intake

Reducing sugar and processed food intake is a crucial step in cancer prevention and overall health improvement. Here are practical strategies to help you make healthier choices:

1. Read Labels:

- **Ingredients:** Learn to read food labels and ingredient lists. Avoid products with added sugars, unhealthy fats, and artificial additives. Look for whole foods with minimal processing.
- **Sugar Content**: Be aware of the different names for sugar (e.g., high-fructose corn syrup, sucrose, glucose) and choose products with low sugar content.

2. Choose Whole Foods:

- **Fresh Produce:** Prioritize fresh fruits and vegetables, which are naturally low in sugar and high in fiber, vitamins, and minerals.
- **Whole Grains:** Opt for whole grains such as brown rice, quinoa, oats, and whole wheat products instead of refined grains.

3. Cook at Home:

- **Homemade Meals:** Preparing meals at home allows you to control the ingredients and avoid hidden sugars and unhealthy fats found in restaurant and pre-packaged foods.

- **Healthy Recipes:** Explore healthy recipes that focus on whole, unprocessed ingredients. Experiment with herbs and spices to enhance flavor without relying on added sugars.

4. Limit Sugary Beverages:

- **Water and Herbal Teas:** Replace sugary drinks like sodas and energy drinks with water, herbal teas, or infused water with slices of fruit for natural sweetness.

- **Fresh Juices:** If you enjoy fruit juices, opt for freshly squeezed juices without added sugars, and consume them in moderation.

5. Smart Snacking:

- **Healthy Snacks:** Choose snacks such as fresh fruits, nuts, seeds, and yogurt instead of processed snacks like chips, cookies, and candy.

- **Portion Control:** Pay attention to portion sizes to avoid overeating, even when choosing healthier snack options.

6. Plan and Prepare:

- **Meal Planning:** Plan your meals and snacks in advance to ensure you have healthy options readily available and reduce the temptation to choose processed foods.
- **Batch Cooking:** Cook large batches of healthy meals and freeze portions for later use. This can save time and help you stick to healthy eating habits.

7. Educate Yourself:

- **Nutrition Knowledge:** Educate yourself about the nutritional content of foods and the impact of different ingredients on your health. Understanding how foods affect your body can motivate you to make better choices.

- **Stay Informed:** Keep up with current research and guidelines on healthy eating and cancer prevention.

Reducing sugar and processed food intake is essential for cancer prevention and overall health. By understanding the impact of these foods on your body, making informed choices, and adopting healthy eating habits, you can significantly lower your cancer risk and improve your quality of life. Emphasize whole, nutrient-dense foods in your diet and be mindful of your sugar and processed food consumption to support long-term health and well-being.

Chapter 6: Practical Tips for a Cancer-Preventive Diet

Adopting a cancer-preventive diet involves more than just knowing which foods are beneficial. It requires practical strategies for meal planning, shopping, cooking, and snacking. This chapter provides detailed guidance to help you integrate cancer-preventive foods into your daily routine effectively.

Creating a Balanced Meal Plan

A balanced meal plan is key to ensuring you get all the nutrients needed for cancer prevention and overall health. Here's how to create a nutritious, balanced meal plan:

1. Emphasize Plant-Based Foods:

- **Fruits and Vegetables:** Aim to fill half your plate with fruits and vegetables at every meal. Choose a variety of colors and types to ensure a wide range of nutrients and phytochemicals.

- **Whole Grains:** Include whole grains such as brown rice, quinoa, oats, and whole wheat products. These provide fiber, which is important for digestive health and cancer prevention.

2. Include Healthy Proteins:

- **Plant-Based Proteins:** Incorporate legumes (beans, lentils, chickpeas), nuts, and seeds as primary protein sources. These foods are rich in fiber, vitamins, and minerals.
- **Lean Animal Proteins:** If you consume animal products, choose lean options such as fish, poultry, and eggs. Fatty fish like salmon and mackerel are excellent sources of omega-3 fatty acids.

3. Incorporate Healthy Fats:

- **Omega-3 Fatty Acids:** Include sources of omega-3s like flaxseeds, chia seeds, walnuts, and fatty fish.
- **Monounsaturated and Polyunsaturated Fats:** Use olive oil, avocado oil, and nuts for cooking

and dressings. Avoid trans fats and limit saturated fats.

4. Limit Red and Processed Meats:

- **Red Meat:** Limit consumption of red meat (beef, pork, lamb) to reduce cancer risk, especially colorectal cancer.
- **Processed Meats**: Avoid processed meats like sausages, hot dogs, and deli meats, which are linked to higher cancer risk.

5. Stay Hydrated:

- **Water:** Make water your primary beverage. It helps maintain bodily functions and can aid in weight management.
- **Herbal Teas:** Herbal teas without added sugars are a good alternative to sugary drinks.

6. Practice Portion Control:

- **Serving Sizes:** Be mindful of portion sizes to avoid overeating. Use smaller plates and bowls to help control portions.

- **Balanced Portions:** Aim for a balance of protein, fiber, and healthy fats at each meal to keep you satisfied and energized.

Shopping for Cancer-Preventive Foods

Shopping smartly is the first step to ensuring you have the right ingredients for a cancer-preventive diet. Here are some tips:

1. Plan Ahead:

- **Meal Planning:** Create a weekly meal plan and shopping list based on healthy recipes. Planning ahead helps you avoid impulse buys and ensures you have all the necessary ingredients.
- **Check Inventory:** Before shopping, check your pantry, refrigerator, and freezer to see what you already have.

2. Shop the Perimeter:

- **Fresh Produce:** Spend most of your time in the produce section, where you'll find fresh fruits and vegetables.
- **Whole Foods:** Focus on whole foods and avoid the inner aisles where processed and packaged foods are typically found.

3. Read Labels:

- **Ingredient Lists**: Read ingredient lists on packaged foods to avoid added sugars, unhealthy fats, and artificial additives.
- **Nutrition Facts:** Check the Nutrition Facts panel for information on serving sizes, calories, and nutrient content.

4. Buy Seasonal and Local:

- **Seasonal Produce:** Buy fruits and vegetables that are in season for better flavor, nutrition, and cost savings.
- **Local Markets:** Shop at farmers' markets to support local agriculture and get fresh, locally grown produce.

5. Choose Organic When Possible:

- **Organic Options:** If possible, choose organic produce to reduce exposure to pesticides. Prioritize organic options for the "Dirty Dozen" (produce with higher pesticide residues) and opt for conventional for the "Clean Fifteen" (produce with lower residues).

Cooking Techniques to Preserve Nutrients

Cooking methods can significantly affect the nutrient content of foods. Here are some techniques to preserve nutrients while preparing cancer-preventive meals:

1. Steaming:

- **Minimal Nutrient Loss:** Steaming vegetables preserves more nutrients compared to boiling. Use a steamer basket over a pot of boiling water and cook until just tender.

2. Roasting and Baking:

- **Flavor and Nutrients:** Roasting and baking can enhance the flavor of vegetables while preserving nutrients. Use moderate temperatures and cook until vegetables are tender but not overcooked.

3. Sautéing and Stir-Frying:

- **Quick Cooking:** Sautéing and stir-frying with a small amount of healthy oil (like olive or avocado oil) is a quick cooking method that retains nutrients. Use high heat for a short time to keep vegetables crisp.

4. Grilling:

- **Healthy Grilling:** Grilling can add a delicious flavor to vegetables and lean proteins. Avoid charring foods, as this can produce harmful compounds. Use marinades with herbs and spices to enhance flavor and add antioxidant properties.

5. Raw and Lightly Cooked:

- **Freshness:** Some vegetables, like leafy greens and cruciferous vegetables, are best consumed

raw or lightly cooked to preserve their
cancer-fighting phytochemicals. Add raw
vegetables to salads or lightly steam them for a
brief time.

6. Blanching:

- **Quick Cook and Cool:** Blanching involves
  briefly boiling vegetables and then plunging them
  into ice water to stop cooking. This method
  preserves color, texture, and nutrients.

Healthy Snacking: Ideas and Recipes

Snacking can be part of a healthy diet if you choose
nutrient-dense options. Here are some healthy snack
ideas and recipes to keep you satisfied between meals:

1. Fresh Fruit:

- **Simple Snacks**: Fresh fruit is a convenient and
  nutritious snack. Apples, bananas, berries, and
  oranges are easy to grab and eat on the go.

- **Fruit Salad:** Combine a variety of fresh fruits for a colorful and nutrient-packed fruit salad. Add a squeeze of lemon or lime juice for extra flavor.

2. Nuts and Seeds:

- **Nut Mix:** Create a homemade nut mix with almonds, walnuts, and pistachios. Add some dried fruit (without added sugar) for natural sweetness.
- **Seed Mix:** Mix pumpkin seeds, sunflower seeds, and chia seeds for a crunchy and nutritious snack.

3. Vegetables and Hummus:

- **Veggie Sticks**: Slice carrots, celery, bell peppers, and cucumbers into sticks. Pair with hummus for a satisfying and fiber-rich snack.
- **Hummus Variations:** Try different flavors of hummus, such as roasted red pepper, garlic, or beet hummus.

4. Greek Yogurt:

- **Toppings:** Top plain Greek yogurt with fresh berries, a drizzle of honey, and a sprinkle of nuts or seeds for added texture and flavor.

- **Smoothies:** Blend Greek yogurt with fruits, spinach, and a bit of flaxseed or chia seeds for a nutritious and creamy smoothie.

5. Whole-Grain Crackers and Avocado:

- **Avocado Toast:** Spread mashed avocado on whole-grain crackers or toast. Sprinkle with salt, pepper, and a squeeze of lemon juice.

- **Guacamole:** Make a simple guacamole with mashed avocado, lime juice, chopped tomatoes, and onions. Use as a dip for whole-grain crackers or vegetable sticks.

6. Energy Bites:

- **No-Bake Bites:** Combine oats, nut butter, honey, and dark chocolate chips in a bowl. Roll into bite-sized balls and refrigerate for a quick, energy-boosting snack.

- **Varieties:** Experiment with different ingredients like dried fruit, coconut flakes, and chia seeds to create your favorite flavor combinations.

7. Dark Chocolate:

- **Antioxidant-Rich:** Choose dark chocolate with at least 70% cocoa for a treat that's rich in antioxidants. Enjoy a small piece with nuts or fruit for a balanced snack.

8. Smoothie Bowls:

- **Base:** Blend frozen berries, a banana, and a splash of almond milk to create a thick smoothie base.
- **Toppings:** Top with granola, fresh fruit, chia seeds, and a drizzle of honey for a nutrient-dense and visually appealing snack.

Practical tips for adopting a cancer-preventive diet include creating a balanced meal plan, smart shopping, using cooking techniques that preserve nutrients, and choosing healthy snacks. By incorporating these strategies into your daily routine, you can enjoy a variety of delicious and nutritious foods that support cancer prevention and overall health. Making mindful choices and being proactive about your diet can have a profound impact on your well-being and long-term health.

Chapter 7: Superfoods for Cancer Prevention

Superfoods are nutrient-rich foods that offer significant health benefits, including cancer prevention. This chapter explores some of the most powerful superfoods and their specific roles in reducing cancer risk.

Turmeric and Curcumin: Anti-Inflammatory Powerhouses

Turmeric, a golden-yellow spice commonly used in Indian cuisine, contains a compound called curcumin, which has been extensively studied for its anti-inflammatory and anti-cancer properties.

Anti-Inflammatory Properties:

- **Curcumin's Role:** Curcumin is the active ingredient in turmeric responsible for its health benefits. It has strong anti-inflammatory effects, which are crucial because chronic inflammation can lead to cancer.

- **Inhibition of Inflammatory Pathways:** Curcumin inhibits various molecules that play a role in inflammation, including nuclear factor-kappa B (NF-κB) and cyclooxygenase-2 (COX-2), both of which are involved in the inflammatory process and are linked to cancer progression.

Antioxidant Effects:

- **Neutralizing Free Radicals:** Curcumin is a potent antioxidant that neutralizes free radicals, which are unstable molecules that can cause DNA damage and contribute to cancer development.

- **Boosting Antioxidant Enzymes:** It also enhances the activity of the body's own antioxidant enzymes, providing a double layer of protection against oxidative stress.

Cancer Cell Growth Inhibition:

- **Apoptosis Induction:** Curcumin can induce apoptosis, or programmed cell death, in cancer cells, preventing their proliferation.

- **Anti-Angiogenesis**: It also inhibits angiogenesis, the formation of new blood vessels that tumors need to grow.

Incorporating Turmeric and Curcumin into Your Diet:

- **Turmeric Powder:** Add turmeric powder to soups, stews, and curries. It pairs well with black pepper, which enhances curcumin absorption.
- **Golden Milk:** Prepare golden milk by mixing turmeric with warm milk (dairy or plant-based), a pinch of black pepper, and a dash of honey.
- **Curcumin Supplements:** For a more concentrated dose, consider curcumin supplements, but consult with a healthcare provider for the appropriate dosage.

Green Tea: Antioxidant-Rich and Health-Boosting

Green tea, made from the leaves of Camellia sinensis, is rich in antioxidants and has been linked to numerous health benefits, including cancer prevention.

Antioxidant Powerhouse:

- **Epigallocatechin Gallate (EGCG):** Green tea contains catechins, with EGCG being the most potent. EGCG has powerful antioxidant properties that protect cells from damage.
- **Oxidative Stress Reduction:** The antioxidants in green tea neutralize free radicals and reduce oxidative stress, which is associated with cancer development.

Anti-Cancer Mechanisms:

- **Cell Cycle Regulation:** EGCG can inhibit the growth of cancer cells by disrupting the cell cycle, preventing them from multiplying.
- **Induction of Apoptosis:** Green tea compounds can induce apoptosis in cancer cells, reducing tumor growth.
- **Inhibition of Metastasis:** Green tea polyphenols may also prevent metastasis, the spread of cancer to other parts of the body, by affecting molecular

pathways involved in cell adhesion and migration.

Incorporating Green Tea into Your Diet:

- **Brewed Tea:** Drink several cups of green tea daily to maximize its health benefits. Avoid adding sugar or sweeteners.
- **Matcha:** Try matcha, a powdered form of green tea, which contains higher concentrations of antioxidants. Use it in teas, lattes, or smoothies.
- **Cooking with Green Tea:** Incorporate green tea into cooking by using it as a base for soups or adding matcha powder to baked goods.

Garlic and Onions: Nature's Antibiotics

Garlic and onions belong to the Allium family and are known for their strong flavors and potent health benefits, including cancer prevention.

Active Compounds:

- **Allicin**: When garlic is chopped or crushed, it produces allicin, a compound with anti-inflammatory, antioxidant, and anti-cancer properties.
- **Sulfur** Compounds: Onions contain sulfur compounds, such as quercetin, which have similar health benefits.

Cancer-Fighting Properties:

- **Detoxification**: Garlic and onions enhance the body's detoxification processes by boosting the production of detoxifying enzymes.
- **Immune Support:** They stimulate the immune system, helping the body to identify and destroy abnormal cells.
- **Anti-Angiogenesis:** These vegetables inhibit angiogenesis, preventing the formation of new blood vessels that supply tumors.

Research Evidence:

- **Epidemiological Studies:** Studies have shown that high consumption of garlic and onions is associated with a reduced risk of several cancers, including stomach, colorectal, and prostate cancers.

- **Laboratory Studies:** Laboratory research indicates that compounds in garlic and onions can inhibit cancer cell growth and induce apoptosis.

Incorporating Garlic and Onions into Your Diet:

- **Raw and Cooked:** Add raw garlic to salads and dressings or cook it in various dishes. Onions can be used in soups, stews, stir-fries, and salads.
- **Garlic Supplements:** For those who dislike the taste of garlic, odorless garlic supplements are available, but consult a healthcare provider for appropriate use.

Berries and Grapes: Rich in Resveratrol and Ellagic Acid

Berries and grapes are not only delicious but also packed with powerful compounds that have anti-cancer properties.

Key Compounds:

- **Resveratrol:** Found in the skin of grapes (especially red grapes), resveratrol is a polyphenol with strong antioxidant and anti-inflammatory effects.
- **Ellagic Acid**: Present in berries such as strawberries, raspberries, and blackberries, ellagic acid has been shown to inhibit cancer cell growth.

Antioxidant and Anti-Inflammatory Properties:

- **Free Radical Neutralization:** Resveratrol and ellagic acid neutralize free radicals, reducing oxidative stress and preventing DNA damage.

- **Inflammation Reduction:** These compounds reduce inflammation, a key factor in cancer development.

Cancer Cell Growth Inhibition:

- **Cell Cycle Arrest:** Resveratrol and ellagic acid can cause cell cycle arrest, stopping cancer cells from dividing.
- **Induction of Apoptosis:** They can also induce apoptosis, leading to the programmed death of cancer cells.

Research Evidence:

- **Laboratory Studies:** Laboratory studies have shown that resveratrol and ellagic acid can inhibit the growth of various cancer cells, including breast, prostate, and colon cancers.
- **Animal Studies:** Animal studies suggest that these compounds can reduce tumor size and prevent metastasis.

Incorporating Berries and Grapes into Your Diet:

- **Fresh and Frozen:** Enjoy fresh berries and grapes as snacks, in salads, or as toppings for yogurt and oatmeal. Frozen berries are a convenient option for smoothies and baking.

- **Juices and Smoothies:** Blend berries and grapes into smoothies or make fresh juice for a nutrient-packed beverage.

- **Dried Fruits:** Dried berries and grapes (raisins) can be added to cereals, trail mixes, and baked goods.

In summary, incorporating superfoods like turmeric, green tea, garlic, onions, berries, and grapes into your diet can significantly contribute to cancer prevention. These foods are rich in compounds that fight inflammation, neutralize free radicals, and inhibit cancer cell growth. By understanding their unique properties and learning how to incorporate them into your daily meals, you can enhance your diet's protective effects and support your long-term health. Embrace these superfoods as part of a balanced, nutritious diet to reduce your cancer risk and improve your overall well-being.

Chapter 8: Supplements and Cancer Prevention

In the quest for optimal health and cancer prevention, many people turn to dietary supplements to ensure they are getting the necessary nutrients. While a balanced diet rich in whole foods is the best way to obtain essential nutrients, supplements can play a role in filling nutritional gaps and providing additional health benefits. This chapter explores when and why to consider supplements, the essential vitamins and minerals for cancer prevention, and safe and effective supplementation practices.

When and Why to Consider Supplements

Nutritional Gaps:

- **Dietary Insufficiencies:** Despite best efforts, it can be challenging to obtain all essential nutrients from diet alone due to factors such as dietary restrictions, food availability, and lifestyle. Supplements can help bridge these gaps.

- **Specific Needs:** Certain life stages and conditions increase nutrient needs, such as pregnancy, aging, illness, or recovery from surgery. Supplements can ensure adequate intake during these times.

Health Conditions:

- **Deficiency Correction**: Supplements can correct specific nutrient deficiencies diagnosed through medical tests, such as iron deficiency anemia or vitamin D deficiency.
- **Chronic Diseases:** Individuals with chronic diseases (e.g., celiac disease, Crohn's disease) may have malabsorption issues, necessitating supplements to maintain adequate nutrient levels.

Cancer Prevention:

- **Enhanced Protection:** Some supplements have been studied for their potential to enhance cancer protection. For example, omega-3 fatty acids, vitamin D, and certain antioxidants may offer additional protective benefits beyond diet alone.

- **High-Risk Individuals:** Those with a family history of cancer or other risk factors may consider targeted supplementation to support overall health and reduce cancer risk.

Essential Vitamins and Minerals for Cancer Prevention

Vitamin D:

Role in Cancer Prevention: Vitamin D is crucial for bone health, immune function, and cell growth regulation. Adequate vitamin D levels have been associated with a lower risk of certain cancers, including colorectal, breast, and prostate cancers.

Sources: Sunlight exposure, fatty fish, fortified foods, and supplements.

Supplementation: Vitamin D3 (cholecalciferol) is the preferred form for supplementation. The recommended dosage varies based on individual needs and blood levels, but common doses range from 1,000 to 2,000 IU per day.

Vitamin C:

Antioxidant Properties: Vitamin C is a powerful antioxidant that protects cells from oxidative damage and supports immune function.

Sources: Citrus fruits, berries, bell peppers, and leafy greens.

Supplementation: Vitamin C supplements are available in various forms, including ascorbic acid, buffered vitamin C, and liposomal vitamin C. Common dosages range from 500 to 1,000 mg per day.

Vitamin E:

Cell Protection: Vitamin E is an antioxidant that protects cell membranes from oxidative damage and may have a role in cancer prevention.

Sources: Nuts, seeds, spinach, and vegetable oils.

Supplementation: Vitamin E supplements are available as alpha-tocopherol. It is important to choose natural forms (d-alpha-tocopherol) rather than synthetic (dl-alpha-tocopherol). Typical doses range from 100 to 400 IU per day.

Selenium:

Cancer Risk Reduction: Selenium is a trace mineral with antioxidant properties that may reduce the risk of certain cancers, particularly prostate cancer.

Sources: Brazil nuts, seafood, meats, and grains.

Supplementation: Selenium supplements are available as selenomethionine or sodium selenite. The recommended daily dose is typically 200 mcg, but it is important not to exceed this amount to avoid toxicity.

Folate (Vitamin B9):

DNA Synthesis and Repair: Folate is essential for DNA synthesis and repair, which is crucial for preventing cancer cell mutations.

Sources: Leafy greens, legumes, nuts, and fortified grains.

Supplementation: Folate is available as folic acid in supplements. The recommended daily dose is typically 400 mcg, but higher doses may be necessary for certain individuals, such as pregnant women.

Omega-3 Fatty Acids:

Anti-Inflammatory Effects: Omega-3 fatty acids have anti-inflammatory properties and may reduce the risk of cancers linked to chronic inflammation, such as colon and breast cancer.

Sources: Fatty fish (salmon, mackerel, sardines), flaxseeds, chia seeds, and walnuts.

Supplementation: Omega-3 supplements are available as fish oil or algal oil (for vegetarians). Typical doses range from 1,000 to 2,000 mg of EPA and DHA combined per day.

Safe and Effective Supplementation Practices

Consultation with Healthcare Providers:

- **Professional Guidance:** Always consult with a healthcare provider before starting any supplement regimen, especially if you have existing health conditions or are taking medications.
- **Personalized Recommendations:** A healthcare provider can offer personalized advice based on your health status, dietary habits, and specific needs.

Quality and Purity:

- **Reputable Brands:** Choose supplements from reputable brands that have undergone third-party testing for quality and purity.
- **Label Reading:** Read labels carefully to understand the ingredients, dosage, and potential allergens.

Appropriate Dosage:

- **Avoid Over-Supplementation:** More is not always better. Taking excessive amounts of certain vitamins and minerals can be harmful and may increase cancer risk. Follow recommended dosages.

- **Daily Intake Monitoring:** Keep track of your total daily intake from both diet and supplements to avoid exceeding safe levels.

Form and Bioavailability:

- **Best Forms:** Some nutrient forms are better absorbed than others. For example, methylcobalamin is a more bioavailable form of vitamin B12 compared to cyanocobalamin.
- **Combining Nutrients:** Some nutrients enhance each other's absorption. For example, taking vitamin D with a meal that contains fat improves its absorption.

Potential Interactions:

- **Medication Interactions:** Be aware of potential interactions between supplements and medications. For instance, vitamin K can interfere with blood thinners like warfarin.

- **Nutrient Interactions:** Certain nutrients can interact with each other. For example, high doses of zinc can interfere with copper absorption.

Monitoring and Adjustments:

- **Regular Testing:** Periodic testing of nutrient levels (e.g., vitamin D, iron) can help monitor your status and adjust supplementation as needed.
- **Symptom Awareness:** Be aware of any side effects or symptoms that may indicate an imbalance, such as nausea, fatigue, or changes in hair and skin health.

Supplements can play a role in cancer prevention by filling nutritional gaps and providing additional health benefits. Essential vitamins and minerals such as vitamin D, C, E, selenium, folate, and omega-3 fatty acids have been linked to reduced cancer risk. Safe and effective supplementation involves consulting healthcare providers, choosing high-quality supplements, adhering to appropriate dosages, and being aware of potential interactions. By incorporating these practices, you can enhance your nutrient intake and support your overall health and well-being.

Chapter 9: Diet Myths and Facts About Cancer Prevention

The relationship between diet and cancer prevention is a topic rife with misinformation and myths. While many claims about "miracle" foods or "cancer-causing" foods abound, it's essential to rely on evidence-based facts to make informed dietary choices. This chapter aims to debunk common myths, present evidence-based facts about diet and cancer risk, and provide guidance on how to stay informed and avoid misinformation.

Debunking Common Myths

Myth 1: Superfoods Can Cure Cancer

The Reality: While certain foods, known as superfoods, contain high levels of nutrients and antioxidants that can help reduce cancer risk, no single food can cure cancer. Cancer prevention and treatment require a holistic approach involving a balanced diet, regular exercise, and medical treatments as needed.

Evidence: Studies show that a diet rich in a variety of fruits, vegetables, whole grains, and lean proteins can contribute to overall health and reduce cancer risk, but they are part of a broader healthy lifestyle.

Myth 2: Sugar Directly Feeds Cancer Cells

The Reality: The claim that sugar directly feeds cancer cells and promotes their growth is an oversimplification. While cancer cells do consume more glucose than normal cells, all cells in the body use glucose for energy. Eliminating sugar entirely is not practical or necessary for cancer prevention.

Evidence: A balanced diet that moderates sugar intake and focuses on complex carbohydrates, such as whole grains, vegetables, and fruits, is recommended. High consumption of sugary foods and beverages should be avoided because they contribute to obesity, which is a risk factor for cancer.

Myth 3: Organic Foods Are Always Better for Cancer Prevention

The Reality: While organic foods are free from synthetic pesticides and fertilizers, there is no conclusive evidence that they are significantly more effective at preventing cancer compared to conventionally grown foods.

Evidence: The most important factor is consuming a diet rich in fruits and vegetables, regardless of whether they are organic or conventionally grown. The nutritional content of organic and conventional foods is generally similar.

Myth 4: Red Meat Always Causes Cancer

The Reality: While there is evidence linking high consumption of red and processed meats to an increased risk of colorectal cancer, moderate consumption of lean red meat as part of a balanced diet can fit into a healthy eating plan.

Evidence: The key is moderation and choosing healthier cooking methods, such as grilling or baking instead of frying, and incorporating a variety of protein sources, including fish, poultry, beans, and legumes.

Myth 5: You Must Follow a Strict, Specific Diet to Prevent Cancer

The Reality: There is no one-size-fits-all diet for cancer prevention. Different dietary patterns, such as the Mediterranean diet, plant-based diets, and others, have been associated with lower cancer risk.

Evidence: The focus should be on overall dietary patterns that emphasize a variety of nutrient-dense foods, portion control, and balanced nutrition. Flexibility in dietary choices allows for a sustainable and enjoyable approach to eating.

Evidence-Based Facts About Diet and Cancer Risk

Fact 1: Fruits and Vegetables Are Crucial for Cancer Prevention

Evidence: Numerous studies have shown that diets high in fruits and vegetables are associated with a lower risk of various cancers. These foods provide essential vitamins, minerals, fiber, and antioxidants that help protect cells from damage.

Recommendation: Aim to fill half your plate with fruits and vegetables at each meal. Include a variety of colors and types to ensure a broad range of nutrients.

Fact 2: Whole Grains Reduce Cancer Risk

Evidence: Whole grains are rich in fiber, which aids in digestion and helps prevent colorectal cancer. They also contain vitamins, minerals, and phytonutrients that contribute to overall health.

Recommendation: Replace refined grains with whole grains such as brown rice, quinoa, whole wheat, and oats. Aim for at least three servings of whole grains per day.

Fact 3: Healthy Fats Are Important

Evidence: Consuming healthy fats, particularly omega-3 fatty acids, has been linked to reduced inflammation and lower cancer risk. Sources include fatty fish, flaxseeds, chia seeds, and walnuts.

Recommendation: Incorporate healthy fats into your diet while limiting saturated and trans fats. Choose sources like olive oil, avocados, and nuts.

Fact 4: Limiting Processed Foods and Red Meat Reduces Cancer Risk

Evidence: High intake of processed foods and red meat has been associated with an increased risk of colorectal cancer. Processed meats contain preservatives and additives that may be carcinogenic.

Recommendation: Limit consumption of processed meats and red meats. Opt for plant-based proteins, fish, and poultry more frequently.

Fact 5: Maintaining a Healthy Weight is Critical

Evidence: Obesity is a significant risk factor for several types of cancer, including breast, colorectal, and pancreatic cancers. Maintaining a healthy weight through diet and exercise is crucial.

Recommendation: Focus on a balanced diet and regular physical activity to achieve and maintain a healthy weight. Monitor portion sizes and avoid high-calorie, low-nutrient foods.

How to Stay Informed and Avoid Misinformation

Follow Reputable Sources:

- **Health Organizations:** Rely on information from reputable health organizations such as the American Cancer Society, World Health Organization, and National Cancer Institute.
- **Medical Journals:** Look for studies and reviews published in reputable medical journals. These sources provide peer-reviewed research and evidence-based recommendations.

Be Skeptical of Miracle Claims:

- **Red Flags:** Be cautious of any diet or product that claims to cure or prevent cancer with little or no evidence. These claims are often not supported by scientific research.
- **Critical Evaluation:** Evaluate the credibility of the source and the evidence provided. Check if

the information is supported by scientific studies and expert opinions.

Consult Healthcare Professionals:

- **Dietitians and Nutritionists:** Seek advice from registered dietitians and nutritionists who specialize in cancer prevention and treatment.
- **Oncologists:** For those diagnosed with cancer, consult oncologists and healthcare providers for personalized dietary recommendations that complement medical treatment.

Stay Updated:

- **Continuing Research:** Nutrition science is continually evolving. Stay informed about new research findings and guidelines by following trusted health news sources and journals.
- **Adapt and Adjust:** Be open to adjusting your diet based on the latest evidence and your personal health needs. What works best for cancer prevention may change as new research emerges.

Avoid Fad Diets:

Balanced Approach: Embrace a balanced and sustainable approach to eating rather than restrictive fad diets. Focus on overall dietary patterns rather than individual foods or nutrients.

Use Technology Wisely:

- **Health Apps:** Utilize reputable health and nutrition apps that provide evidence-based information and tools to track your diet and health metrics.
- **Online Communities:** Engage in online communities and forums that are moderated by healthcare professionals. These can be valuable for support and information sharing.

Understanding the facts about diet and cancer prevention is essential for making informed decisions about your health. By debunking common myths, relying on evidence-based information, and staying informed, you can adopt a diet that supports your overall well-being and reduces your cancer risk. Remember that a balanced diet rich in fruits, vegetables, whole grains, and healthy fats, combined with regular physical activity and weight management, is the cornerstone of cancer prevention.

Chapter 10: Integrating a Cancer-Preventive Diet into Your Lifestyle

Adopting a cancer-preventive diet is not just about what you eat; it's about embracing a lifestyle that supports long-term health and well-being. This chapter explores strategies for overcoming challenges, staying motivated, gaining family and social support, and reaping the long-term benefits of a cancer-preventive diet.

Overcoming Challenges and Staying Motivated

Identifying Barriers:

- **Time Constraints:** Busy schedules can make meal planning and preparation challenging. However, prioritizing health can lead to more efficient and productive days.
- **Budget Concerns:** Healthy eating can be perceived as expensive, but with careful planning, it can be affordable. Buying in bulk, opting for seasonal produce, and cooking at home can help save money.

- **Cravings and Temptations:** Unhealthy foods may be tempting, especially in social settings or during stressful times. Finding healthier alternatives and practicing mindful eating can help overcome these challenges.

Setting Realistic Goals:

- **Short-Term Goals:** Set achievable goals, such as adding one extra serving of vegetables to your meals each day or trying a new cancer-preventive recipe each week.
- **Long-Term Goals:** Aim for long-term changes, such as maintaining a balanced diet, regular physical activity, and a healthy weight, which can significantly reduce cancer risk over time.

Tracking Progress:

- **Food Diary:** Keep a food diary to track your meals, snacks, and water intake. This can help you identify patterns, track progress, and stay accountable.

- **Health Metrics:** Monitor your health metrics, such as weight, cholesterol levels, and blood pressure, to track improvements and stay motivated.

Rewarding Yourself:

- **Non-Food Rewards:** Celebrate your successes with non-food rewards, such as a relaxing bath, a new book, or a movie night. This can reinforce positive behaviors and motivate you to stay on track.

Family and Social Support: Getting Everyone on Board

Leading by Example:

- **Family Influence:** Engage your family in meal planning and preparation. Encourage them to try new cancer-preventive foods and recipes.

- **Social Support:** Share your goals with friends and family. Their support and encouragement can help you stay motivated and accountable.

Educating Your Circle:

- **Sharing Information**: Share evidence-based information about cancer prevention and the benefits of a healthy diet with your family and friends. This can help them understand and support your dietary choices.

Creating a Supportive Environment:

- **Healthy Options:** Keep your home stocked with cancer-preventive foods, making it easier to make healthy choices.
- **Mindful Eating:** Practice mindful eating during family meals, focusing on the flavors and textures of your food. This can help you savor your meals and prevent overeating.

Long-Term Benefits and Sustaining Healthy Habits

Reduced Cancer Risk:

- **Long-Term Impact:** Embracing a cancer-preventive diet can significantly reduce your risk of developing various types of cancer, as well as other chronic diseases.
- **Improved Overall Health:** In addition to cancer prevention, a healthy diet can lead to weight management, better heart health, improved digestion, and increased energy levels.

Sustainability:

- **Lifestyle Change:** View your dietary changes as a long-term lifestyle change rather than a short-term diet. This mindset shift can help you sustain healthy habits over time.
- **Flexibility:** Allow for flexibility in your diet. Occasional indulgences or deviations from your usual routine are normal and should not derail your overall progress.

Positive Impact on Future Generations:

- **Setting an Example:** By adopting a cancer-preventive diet, you are setting a positive example for your children and future generations. Your healthy habits can inspire those around you to prioritize their health.

Quality of Life:

- **Enhanced Well-Being:** A diet rich in cancer-preventive foods can improve your overall well-being, including mood, cognitive function, and quality of life.

Embracing a Holistic Approach:

- **Physical Activity:** Incorporate regular physical activity into your routine, as it complements a healthy diet in reducing cancer risk.
- **Stress Management:** Practice stress-reducing techniques such as mindfulness, yoga, or meditation. Chronic stress can contribute to inflammation and increase cancer risk.

Regular Health Check-ups:

- **Monitoring Health:** Schedule regular check-ups with your healthcare provider to monitor your health and discuss any concerns or changes in your diet or lifestyle.

Incorporating a cancer-preventive diet into your lifestyle is a proactive step towards reducing your cancer risk and improving your overall health. By overcoming challenges, staying motivated, gaining family and social support, and focusing on the long-term benefits, you can make sustainable changes that enhance your well-being. Remember, every small step towards a healthier lifestyle counts, and the journey is as important as the destination. Embrace the process, stay positive, and celebrate your progress along the way.

Conclusion: Your Path to a Healthier, Cancer-Free Life

Congratulations on taking the proactive step towards reducing your cancer risk and improving your overall health through a cancer-preventive diet! By incorporating the principles outlined in this book into your lifestyle, you are on the path to a healthier, cancer-free life. In this concluding chapter, we'll recap the key points discussed throughout the book, help you create a personal action plan, and provide resources for further reading and support.

Recap of Key Points

Nutrient-Rich Diet: A diet rich in fruits, vegetables, whole grains, lean proteins, and healthy fats provides essential nutrients and antioxidants that help protect against cancer.

Phytochemicals and Antioxidants: Phytochemicals and antioxidants found in plant-based foods have been shown to have cancer-preventive properties.

Healthy Fats: Omega-3 fatty acids and other healthy fats play a role in reducing inflammation and lowering cancer risk.

Limiting Sugars and Processed Foods: High intake of sugars and processed foods should be avoided, as they can contribute to inflammation and increase cancer risk.

Supplements: While a balanced diet is the best way to obtain nutrients, supplements can be beneficial for filling nutritional gaps, especially in high-risk individuals or those with specific dietary needs.

Lifestyle Factors: In addition to diet, maintaining a healthy weight, staying physically active, managing stress, and avoiding tobacco and excessive alcohol consumption are important for cancer prevention.

Creating a Personal Action Plan

1. Assess Your Current Diet: Keep a food diary for a week to understand your current eating habits and identify areas for improvement.

2. Set Realistic Goals: Based on your assessment, set your achievable goals for incorporating more cancer-preventive foods into your diet and reducing intake of unhealthy foods.

3. Plan Your Meals: Use meal planning to ensure you have nutritious meals and snacks readily available. Include a variety of fruits, vegetables, whole grains, and lean proteins.

4. Stay Active: Incorporate regular physical activity into your routine. Aim for at least 150 minutes of moderate-intensity exercise per week.

5. Manage Stress: Practice stress-reducing techniques such as yoga, meditation, or deep breathing exercises to manage stress, which can contribute to inflammation and cancer risk.

6. Seek Support: Share your goals with friends and family. Their support can help you stay motivated and accountable.

7. Monitor Your Progress: Regularly review your goals and track your progress. Celebrate your successes and adjust your plan as needed.

Resources for Further Reading and Support

- **American Cancer Society (ACS):** Provides information on cancer prevention, early detection, treatment, and support programs. Website: cancer.org
- **National Cancer Institute (NCI):** Offers a wealth of information on cancer research, clinical trials, and cancer prevention. Website: cancer.gov
- **World Cancer Research Fund (WCRF):** Provides evidence-based recommendations for cancer prevention, including diet and lifestyle factors. Website: wcrf.org
- **Local Cancer Support Groups:** Joining a local cancer support group can provide additional support and resources for individuals affected by cancer.

- **Consult a Registered Dietitian:** A registered dietitian can provide personalized advice and support for incorporating a cancer-preventive diet into your lifestyle.

In conclusion, adopting a cancer-preventive diet and lifestyle is a powerful way to reduce your cancer risk and improve your overall health. By making informed dietary choices, staying active, managing stress, and seeking support, you can take control of your health and enjoy a healthier, cancer-free life. Remember, every small change you make towards a healthier lifestyle counts, so keep moving forward on your journey to better health!